Get Your H

Get Your Health Back

How to Feel Better, Reverse Chronic Conditions, and Reclaim Your Mojo

Laura F. Robin, DO, MPH

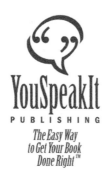

YouSpeakIt

PUBLISHING

The Easy Way to Get Your Book Done Right ™

This book is dedicated to my parents,
Phyllis and Dr. Murray Robin, who selflessly, heartfully,
and humorously gave me every bit of encouragement, support,
and mentoring that I needed to make my dreams happen.

Contents

Acknowledgments

I'd like to thank each of you—from my high school teachers to my college professors to my good friends—who has pushed me past my limits.

I would like to thank my countless mentors from medical school, public health school, and in my osteopathic, integrative, and functional medicine studies. I especially want to thank the pioneers in medicine and functional medicine who had the foresight and courage to lead the rest of us on this path.

Many thanks to my family, and especially to my son, Ari, for putting up with my absences while I have pursued my passion for this work.

Thank you to our past and present team at Rosa Transformational Health for giving our program its outstanding quality.

And most of all, I'd like to thank all my patients who have taught me so much over the years and have had the courage to find a better way.

Introduction

Most people I talk to aren't feeling as well as they would like to feel, and most of these people don't think there is anything they can do about it.

Many people just accept the slow onset of worsening fatigue, foggier brains, increasing pain and stiffness, gut issues, or worsening mood issues as their *new normal*.

We complain to our doctors who tell us that nothing is wrong, or that our symptoms are a normal part of aging.

Those of us who have been diagnosed with chronic medical conditions are told that our medical issues will never get better; they will just get worse, and there is nothing we can do about it.

This book was written for you.

This book was written to expose the truth about our bodies and our health.

Why do so many of us feel so poorly?

What is causing so many of us to feel sub-par?

Is *chronic disease* really forever and progressive?

Is there actually a way to feel better, reverse chronic health problems, and get more out of life?

I was trained in traditional Western medicine, and I have worked in medicine for over thirty years. I have made it my life's work to find ways to help people meet their health goals. I most definitely see the value in what we call "traditional Western Medicine." However, it has become abundantly clear that this type of medicine, which has become so dominant in our culture, is extremely limited and often misses the mark in how it can help people to really get to the root of what is going on in their health and turn it around.

Our healthcare system in the United States excels in some ways. For example, there is no place I would rather be if I had a car accident, was having a heart attack, or needed emergency surgery than at the door of my favorite emergency room in this country. Or, maybe your doctor has prescribed medications to help with symptoms of pain or depression or sleeplessness or has given you medications to help lower your blood sugar or blood pressure or cholesterol. But it has become apparent to me over the years that, although my patients have this emergency help available to them, as well as access to many doctors and medications to relieve symptoms, their day-to-day lives are still very much impaired.

What does this mean?

Here are some indications of an impaired day-to-day life:

- You are not sleeping well, or you are tired all the time.
- Your body hurts.
- Your brain is foggy.

- You feel depressed, or you just don't feel like yourself anymore.
- You rely on one or more toxic medications to make it through your day.
- You look at yourself in the mirror and don't like what you see.
- You are unhappy with your weight or body condition.

If you can relate to any of these items, either from your own experience, or that of a loved one, I have written this book for you. If you have tried to help yourself and have had little to no success, I want to let you know that there is a solution. You do not need to accept that this is your future. You can optimize the way your body functions and the way you feel every day from when you wake up to when you go to bed.

Each of us only has one body in this lifetime, and that body is here to help us to do the things we need and want to do. If your body and your brain aren't working properly, then you will not be able to get to where you want to go to manifest your dreams, your goals, and your purpose in life.

I wrote this book because I am passionate about sending this message out. During my years in practice, I have witnessed too many people suffering for too long, losing hope as time passes. So many people feel like there is nothing they can do about their health but watch it deteriorate.

We in this country are aware of increasing health problems but our response has been to build more assisted-living facilities, more memory-care centers, more surgery centers, and more treatment centers. Meanwhile, our population continues to grow sicker and sicker.

I had blinders on as I went through medical school, which is typical for a traditionally trained medical doctor. My blinders told me that I was limited to using only certain ways to diagnose and treat my patients. I found myself working often—*too* often—with people who were at the end of their rope. It was frustrating and disheartening that so much of my effort was going into treating people who were at the end of their trajectory of failing health. I knew that there must be a way to help prevent people from arriving at this end-stage place.

I started searching. I studied public health and preventive medicine. I became a medical epidemiologist to help to work on the population level with respect to some of these illnesses. I also came to understand the enormous impact that our environment and lifestyle has on how our bodies work.

It also became clear that each of our bodies is unique in how we respond to:

- Environment
- Lifestyle
- Food choices
- Medical treatments

In this book, we will explore many different factors that impact our health, including what we eat, what our bodies are exposed to, and how we deal with the stressors in our lives.

In my search, I have found a different way of looking at what is going on in our bodies. This way is not at all new. It is actually found at the roots of modern Western medicine. It lies in the anatomy, physiology, biochemistry, and cell biology of what is going on in the deepest parts of our bodies. It is there that we can get answers about the root cause of what is happening in our bodies. It is there that we can find out what makes us tired and sick and in pain and not able to function in the world.

Finally, I have found a better way to treat patients. I have joined thousands of doctors around the country who combine their knowledge of modern Western medicine with *Root Cause, or Functional Medicine* to work with their patients and help their patients to optimize their lives, their health, and what they are able to do in the world.

One example is my patient, Jeff, 50, who basically said it all when he and his wife walked into my office for the first time and he proclaimed, "Doc, I lost my Mojo." The slang of the word MOJO means "charm or luck or magic, or the ability to attract beautiful women". It comes from the Portuguese word *molho*, which means "sauce with varying levels of spice". Jeff's loss of mojo included weight gain, loss of muscle mass, loss of libido, low level depressive moods, foggy brain, lack of motivation, and fatigue. He was trying to eat what he thought was a healthy diet and he was exercising. These things were helping a bit, but he just couldn't break through what was keeping him down. Does this sound familiar? (See Conclusion for the follow-up to Jeff's story.)

I have written this book to teach you more about how your body works and to introduce you to these new concepts of health. My goal is to give you the knowledge you need so you can take action and get your health to where you want it to be. I have tried to make it a quick and easy read, so you can quickly start applying what you learn.

After reading this book, it is my hope that you will see that feeling poorly is not normal and feeling better is not out of your grasp—in fact, feeling a lot better is actually quite attainable for most people. I see it on a daily basis. I hope it gives you the motivation to get your health back and reclaim your mojo!

CHAPTER ONE

You Don't Have to Feel Sick

WE ARE LIVING LONGER, BUT WE'RE FEELING WORSE

We in the United States are effectively part of a big experiment. Every person living in the United States is like a subject in an experiment because we all live in an environment that has changed dramatically in the last hundred years.

Many of these changes are positive. We are living longer lives because we have improved sanitation, emergency medications, and emergency surgeries.

Have you, or someone you know, experienced a second or third chance at life because you were saved by emergency treatment, antibiotics, or surgery?

This has definitely been a big advantage of the miracles of modern medicine. However, what happens in those *bonus* years has made many of us downright miserable!

Although we live longer, the reality is that most adults and many children don't actually feel well, and most of the time, we chalk it up to the fact that we are the same as everyone else around us—we assume that it is normal.

For example, many of my patients have come in telling me that they feel tired all the time. They say they have no stamina, they are not sleeping, their mood is low, their brain is foggy, and they *don't feel like themselves* anymore. Their doctor has told them that they are *normal*. Then, they come to me for another opinion.

Doctors have heard so many of these complaints that they may have become desensitized as well. When you tell your doctor how you feel, you may be told that it is, indeed, perfectly normal. In my opinion, and from what I have seen in my practice, it is not.

The Normalization of Feeling Bad

Have you ever heard the old story of the frog in boiling water?

A frog in water at room temperature is very happy. If you put a frog in boiling water, this would not be the case! However, if you start with room temperature water, and heat it slowly, the story goes that the frog won't try to get out. It won't notice the temperature change, and it will eventually die because of the extreme heat of the water.

The story may not be scientifically accurate, but it can be used to illustrate something true about people. We don't usually notice the effects of gradual changes in our environment or our health.

This is, in my opinion, what is happening in the United States. Our norms are changing. It has become normal not to feel well. It has become normal to complain to our healthcare providers and be given another medication. It has become normal to be on multiple medications. We are the most heavily medicated country in the world.

Are these medications taking away our problems?

In the vast majority of cases, no.

Are they going to keep us from getting worse?

In the vast majority of cases, no.

Are they going to turn around the underlying cause of our problems?

Likely not.

Illness in the United States

In America, we have normalized feeling bad. We have also normalized the increase we're seeing in long-term and chronic disorders in our population.

For example, there have been substantial increases in the following conditions:

- Obesity

- Diabetes
- Autoimmune diseases
- Intestinal disorders
- Food and other allergies and sensitivities
- Alzheimer's, Dementia, and foggy brain
- Thyroid and other hormonal imbalances.

We continue to identify new illnesses—like chronic fatigue and fibromyalgia—and we have seen recent increases in the incidence of diseases like chronic Epstein-Barr and Lyme disease. Chronic fatigue and fibromyalgia are both increasing at an alarming rate, as are other autoimmune diseases, like Hashimoto's thyroiditis, lupus, multiple sclerosis, celiac disease, and other autoimmune gastrointestinal illnesses. More children have allergies and asthma than ever before, and our kids are going to school feeling more tired and more stressed than they ever have.

We have some of the best-trained doctors in the world, and most of them have good hearts and the best of intentions. Most doctors want to go into practice because they really care about people and they want to help them. They want to do good in the world. In spite of this, in health ratings, we in the United States rank very low among the industrialized countries. For example, when we compare ourselves to thirty-five countries that have similar levels of medical education and technology, we are ranked thirty-first in life expectancy and twenty-ninth in infant mortality (World Health Organization, 2016)[1]

The Business of Disability

If you have any question about whether our population is becoming sicker and needing more help, you can just look at what is happening in our economy. One of the fastest growing industries is the health industry. This growth includes the building of hospitals, surgery centers, assisted living facilities, and memory-care centers. All kinds of facilities are cropping up to help people who are either unable to take care of themselves or who have these illnesses and disorders that are becoming so much more common.

We should ask ourselves what is going on here. If the health industry is one of the fastest-growing industries in the country, it follows that the economy is in many ways dependent on us *staying sick*.

Do Americans really need this type of assistance or is this growth happening primarily because entrepreneurs can make so much money in this field?

It may look like Americans are truly in need of this type of assistance because we are becoming sicker and sicker. It may seem like there is no other solution. However, this isn't

---

1 *World Health Statistics 2016: Monitoring health for the SDGs Annex B: tables of health statistics by country, WHO region and globally.* World Health Organization. 2016. Retrieved 27 June 2016.

the whole story. *Most people don't know that it doesn't have to be this way.* The truth is that we are not seeing the bigger picture.

Here is some of what we're missing:

- We are not paying attention to what is the underlying cause, or root, of these health problems.

- Unlike what most people believe, it is not inevitable or normal to be in poor health—it has become the norm, but it is *not* normal!

- We are not understanding the fact that most of the illnesses that are increasing in prevalence and incidence can be turned around. These health trends in our population don't have to continue the way they are going.

- Our focus needs shifting—away from the business of building more facilities, prescribing more medications, doing more surgery—to the business of preventing and reversing disease.

NORMAL, NORMAL, NORMAL

We go to our healthcare providers with a lot of complaints that indicate our bodies and brains just aren't working as well as they used to. When I first went into medicine, I was trained as a traditional Western medicine family practice doc. I heard many people come in with what we call common complaints—we'll describe some of them for you in the section below. Over time, I started to become increasingly *deaf* to these common complaints.

I became more and more unable to hear my patients for two reasons. First, I would hear the same complaints so frequently—over and over again—that my mind became acclimated to them, so I essentially stopped paying attention to them. Second, a part of me stopped listening because I knew I wasn't able to do anything about these complaints in the long run.

I think this is an issue with many healthcare providers in the United States today. As caring as they are, when they don't have the answers, it's difficult to keep paying attention—to continue to want to hear about a persistent multitude of problems. They see these issues so frequently that the symptoms are perceived as *normal*.

The word *Disease* **comes from the word roots** *dis-*, **meaning "lack of," and** *ease*: **lack of ease.**

Modern medicine has used the word *disease* to give names, or diagnoses, to groups of signs, symptoms, or lab values.

When we give a group of symptoms a name, we can categorize and study it further. We can isolate it from other diseases so that we can further focus on it. We can then separate it from other things going on in the body so that we can treat it. Some physicians become specialists and sub-specialists in treating certain types of diseases, such as diabetes, kidney failure, and cancer, etc.

The term *dis-ease* gives us an opportunity to look more generally at what is going on. The body is literally not-at-ease. There is a lack of ease in our body. We may or may not have a diagnosis, or we may have several; sometimes we know that certain symptoms are coming from certain diseases that have been found in us. But the term dis-ease is important because it describes what we are feeling and what is happening in our body when we look at it as a whole, and not just the parts with diagnoses.

For example, a *disease* might be:

- Diabetes
- Hashimoto's thyroiditis
- Irritable bowel syndrome
- Fibromyalgia
- Chronic fatigue
- Cancer

Another way of considering what is happening in the body is to put it in the context of *dis-ease,* or:

- Low energy
- Joint or muscle pain

- Foggy brain
- Gastrointestinal symptoms
- Sleep or mood issues
- Weight gain

Some of the Symptoms

When do you go to the doctor?

Certainly, you would go to your doctor if you had intense pain, or if you broke a leg. You would go if you had a terrible respiratory infection or pneumonia. We go to our doctors when we are having a crisis. Our doctors are typically able to give us what we need so that we can get better and feel better in those circumstances.

Modern medicine first evolved when most health problems were acute, or at a crisis level. Doctors were needed to treat serious infections, or to do an emergency surgery like remove an appendix, or to save someone from a traumatic injury.

Over the past fifty to seventy years, the health in our country has changed. Although we still have these emergencies, the bulk of what we go to our doctors for is long-term, or chronic, illness.

We have seen unprecedented epidemics of all kinds of chronic disease, like obesity, heart disease, stroke, cancer, diabetes, autoimmune syndromes, dementia, and pain syndromes. Doctors have specialized and further specialized in the treatments of these conditions.

And the way doctors have evolved medicine to treat these conditions is through two basic means:

1. Drugs
2. Surgery

Modern medicine includes more and more research to find the better surgery and the better drug.

The true answers to actually *treating* and *fixing* our problems are almost completely ignored. Modern medicine just invents another drug to help more effectively with stabilizing blood sugar or a better surgery to replace or fix organs that are failing.

So, our doctors keep treating us for our disease. We get more and more drugs and more and more surgery. But the reality is that for most of us these drugs and surgery are only of temporary and limited help.

Or maybe we don't even have a diagnosis so we can't get a treatment.

Another way in which modern medicine fails us is when we go to the doctor with symptoms that don't fall into a specific disease diagnosis.

These include complaints like:

- Being very tired
- Waking up tired in the morning
- Hitting a wall in the afternoon
- Not being able to fall asleep at night or stay asleep
- Having to get up many times in the night to go to the bathroom
- Chronic or intermittent diarrhea or constipation
- Heartburn or other digestive issues
- Forgetfulness, or an inability to think clearly—what I like to call *brain fog*
- Chronic pain, in our joints or muscles, or nerve pain
- Recent changes in weight that are unexplained
- Weight gained in the last few years that the patient has not been able to lose
- Changes in mood or motivation, or not feeling like yourself anymore

Are You About to Die? Tests

When we go to the doctor complaining of these issues, there are a couple of things going on behind the scenes. First, most of our doctors are feeling rushed all the time. This isn't because they want to move as many people through the office as they can; it's because they need to.

With what has happened in recent years in the medical industry and in the insurance industry, doctors don't usually have control over how much time they are allowed to spend with patients. Even if they do have that control, they have so many expenses and so many requirements that are given to them by the insurance companies that they are forced to move people through more quickly. This makes for a frustrated doctor as well as a frustrated patient. *Everyone* is frustrated.

When you go to the doctor, you may have already had to wait to get an appointment, and then, you may have had to sit a while in the waiting room before you are seen. You may have a whole list of things you want to talk about when you finally get in the exam room. For the practitioner, once your complaints number more than two or three, it often becomes a bit overwhelming—it may be a struggle for the doctor to be able to adequately address all your needs in the amount of time given.

Doctors in this country have a standardized way of looking at your health. Simplistically, this is because each complaint must be given an accompanying diagnosis. Each diagnosis must be given a treatment. If there is no treatment, there might be a referral to another doctor or another test. All of this takes time.

As a result, you are typically asked to pick your top two to four priorities.

It is all an unfortunate symptom of a broken system.

When you complain about a symptom, there is a standard blood evaluation that a doctor may order for you. Usually it is a standard set of tests, called a complete blood count, or CBC, and a Comprehensive Medical Panel, or CMP. A doctor may choose to add another test—to take a quick look at how a patient's thyroid is doing, for instance.

Don't get me wrong. This is an excellent set of tests; they are gold standard and necessary. They tell us a lot about the major functions in our bodies. But they are also very basic. I like to call them the *Are You About to Die?* tests because they really are screening tests to see if you have the big issues like diabetes, kidney failure, or liver disease.

When Tests Come Back Normal

When you go to the doctor with some of these nebulous complaints, the doctor will do these *Are You About to Die?* tests, and often, the test results will come back normal. The doctor, given the amount of time they have, is in essence doing a triage to see if you have something that needs immediate attention—something that could be of immediate danger to your life.

Usually, when the tests come back normal, the doctor is going to tell you that all is well—your kidneys aren't failing, you don't have any big thyroid disease, and you don't have diabetes—and they will be happy about that because many have the sense that their job is to save you from disaster. Having normal blood tests helps them to assure you that there don't appear to be any disasters coming or happening.

They feel like they have done their job because they have not found anything that medically needs immediate treatment.

But the reality is that when you walk out of the office, you are still feeling the way you were feeling when you came in. You still don't have any answers. Many times, that is where your doctor's visit ends. You hoped the doctor would dig farther, but in reality, many doctors will likely feel that they have done their job. They have done what they know they are supposed to do, and they have done it well.

I'm not writing this book to say bad things about your healthcare provider, who you may love and respect. Your doctor may be well trained in the field that they're in and are doing their best. They are very good at taking care of broken bones and broken hearts and broken blood sugar. Your doctor may be the exact person you will need in the future if you were to have a health crisis. However, their training and their system of medicine may fall short of being able to care for what's really happening with you. They may be failing to uncover what's making you feel horrible because they aren't seeing what is happening on a subtler level in your body. You may need to seek a *root-cause* or functional medicine clinician to help you dig deeper and in a different way than your traditional Western doctors are trained or willing to go.

THE WALKING WOUNDED

Early on, when I was in my traditional medical practice, I came to realize that there were a lot of problems that my patients were describing for which I had no answers. These were the patients that I called the walking wounded.

The walking wounded are people who may be able to get up in the morning, get appropriately cleaned up and dressed, and get themselves out in the world. They may be able to work a full day, take care of their children and grandchildren, and do their errands. Nobody would know that there is anything wrong, but inside, they are feeling exhausted, stressed, in pain, and completely out of balance.

Internally Struggling

Since I chose to start working more with the walking wounded, I found that an enormous number of people are out there really struggling each and every day. They are feeling tired, in pain—terribly out of balance. Many of you are feeling that way, but have become convinced that it's *normal*—either because you have already been to a doctor who has told you so, or because you see that your friends and family around you are feeling the same way too. You feel like the way you feel is normal and inevitable—this is just the way it has to be.

We Chalk It Up to Being Normal

Below is a common scenario faced by the walking wounded. See if any of it sounds familiar to you:

You have symptoms that make you feel poorly, but it seems like everyone around you has symptoms too. For example, you are tired, but everyone around you says they feel tired too. You have become forgetful and your body aches, but other people tell you that's to be expected at your age. If you can get through your day, can still work or manage your daily tasks, this is more evidence that how you feel is normal.

When you talk about how you feel, you may be told:

- *Well, you are not a spring chicken anymore.*

- *You're not twenty anymore, so you shouldn't expect to feel the way you did back then.*

- *Everybody's tired; nobody has the energy they did when they were kids.*

- *Aches and pains come with the territory.*

- *Forgetfulness is normal at your age.*

- *Everyone gains weight as they get older—or after they have kids—or at menopause. That is just what happens. It's normal.*

You continue to work and do your daily tasks but wonder if this is really the way you're supposed to feel. Finally, you go to the doctor and ask for help. After a quick visit, your doctor takes some blood, and you are told that your tests are normal.

Then you must be normal, right?

That's just the way it is, right?

Even when you go to a specialist and get more specific testing done, this doesn't guarantee an end to your problems. If you have heartburn or gut issues, you may be told that everything is normal after you've had a normal colonoscopy and other tests with a normal result. You may have major sleep problems, but a sleep study shows that you don't have sleep apnea, so you may be told there is nothing else that the doctor can do.

When the doctor doesn't find the root cause of a problem, he or she may prescribe medications that address the symptoms. For example, if you have sleep problems, you may be prescribed pills to help you sleep. If you are depressed or anxious, you may be given medication. If you have pain, you may be given anti-inflammatories. If you have focus issues, you may be given medications to help you with focus. If you have diarrhea or constipation or heartburn, you may be given medications for those. Medications may work to some extent but do nothing to address the cause of your symptom. Even worse, many of these medications come with terrible side effects or long-term consequences. They also might be very expensive and inconvenient to continue for the rest of your life. And you may require more and more at higher and higher doses in order to maintain effectiveness.

Grin and Bear It

We feel poorly, but look around us and see that so many others are struggling in the same way. We are told that there isn't anything we can do about it, and we go to our doctor only to hear the same thing.

Over time, in our population, we've pretty much normalized the fact that our bodies and brains don't work the way we want them to. Because we are connected with doctors and a healthcare system, we might initially turn to them. We hope that there might be something we can do about how we feel, but after the trip to the doctor, or maybe repeated trips to many doctors, we learn that there really is no hope of feeling any better. Our conclusion is that we just need to grin and bear it.

There is good reason for that. Between the normalization of how we feel and the normalization of how everybody else is feeling, the expectations of the health industry, what we hear on television, and what our doctors tell us, we are going to stop looking, lose hope, and feel like all our maladies are completely normal.

Off the Couch

Karen H. was sixty-nine years old and a retired teacher. Karen came in because she had absolutely no energy and she knew that her health and her life were out of control. About a year before, she had adopted two boys she had been fostering, ages ten and fourteen. She was finding herself so incredibly exhausted that the only thing she had time for was taking care of their basic care needs and nothing else. So, she would wake up in the morning, make their breakfast and make their lunches for school. As soon as they left for school, she would fall asleep on the couch.

Karen would be on the couch until an hour or so before they came home, and she would drag herself up to be able to do what she needed to do with them for the rest of the day. She knew that was completely unsustainable for her. She had diabetes that was out of control, and she had recently consulted with a doctor who was trying to get her to go on insulin. She had severe brain fog and was not able to think clearly. She also had a chronic, low-level cough.

She began our program and within two weeks had pretty much turned around her fatigue. Her blood sugars came into almost immediate control and she never had to go on the insulin. Her energy improved and she started losing weight. Her brain fog completely disappeared, and she was thinking clearly again. She continued to gain energy and was also passing her healthy habits on to her kids, who also benefitted from them.

In the fourth week of the program, she realized that a chronic, low-level cough she had lived with forever had gone away. She realized it was due to sensitivity to a common food that she had been eating daily. Incidentally, she had never even mentioned her cough to me in her intake appointment because there were so many other issues that were more pressing. I see her now only every few months. Her blood sugar is in beautiful control without medications. She is active, happy, and feels very much alive.

Testimonials

I was seventy when I came to Dr. Laura's practice. I know I am going to live past one hundred. It is better to feel good instead of being decrepit. At seventy, I was feeling decrepit. I decided to change that. I lost thirty-five pounds and another five since. I can outrun people who drink coffee. I notice my body functions better.

~ Lauren Jontel, 70, Grandmother,
Caregiver, and Healer

I had been having a lot of pain, [in the back of my leg] for several years. No doctor seemed to think it was anything important, but it hurt to get out of bed, and it restricted my life. I was also constantly exhausted. I am pain free most of the time. My energy is better. My weight is down.

~ Rachel Barrett, 59, Administrator

I came to Rosa Transformational Health because I just felt so bad every day. I would wake up and my stomach would hurt. My knees would hurt. I had no energy and I thought: **there has got to be more to life than this.** *After about four months in the program, I have lost forty pounds and I have tremendous energy. If you have any question about* *not feeling good or not having enough energy, I really encourage you to see what Rosa Transformational Health can do for you because they are awesome!*

~ Karen Hatfield, 69, Retired Teacher
and Newly Adoptive Parent

CHAPTER TWO

Traditional Medicine Versus What I Do

THE LIMITED TOOLBOX

When I was in medical school, I remember being excited because I was learning so many interesting things. I took courses in anatomy, physiology, biochemistry, immunology, microbiology, and cell biology. I learned how our bodies function at levels as deep as we knew to go. The human body is so complex; there are many different moving parts and many things happening, both on levels we can see and on levels we can't see.

The body is fascinating. Its ability to heal itself is unbelievable. Just think about how your body heals itself from a cut or a bruise or a fracture. During medical school, I was excited to learn how I could work with the body to help people get better. I would be able to help them heal from their injuries and illnesses. I was so excited to put all my knowledge into practice!

I began my clinical studies, working under supervising doctors, and I was quickly disappointed. I found that I had to put aside nearly everything I had learned. In addition, I had only a limited—very limited—toolbox to work with.

The Idea of Diagnosis

I chose to go to an osteopathic medical school. Osteopathic medicine, although it gives a DO degree rather than an MD degree, is equivalent in all ways to MD medical schools and produces doctors who have identical privileges. The philosophy of Osteopathy is a little different, however, in its strong belief that everything in our bodies is interconnected, everything effects everything else, and that the person needs to be looked at and treated as a whole, and not just the sum of their parts.

I loved that philosophy, as it always made such sense. However, when I started to see patients in actual practice, the modern medical model I was needing to fit into felt quite incongruent with that philosophy.

I had been so excited to put that philosophy and all my new knowledge of anatomy, biochemistry, and physiology into use! When I started to see patients, however, everything shifted into a different gear.

Here is what I learned during the initial days of my clinical training:

- I had a very limited amount of time to spend with these patients.

- I needed to come up with a diagnosis to satisfy the insurance companies.

- The diagnosis was also necessary because it told me specifically how I needed to treat that patient.

- Each diagnosis had a specific protocol of treatments that went along with it. I call this *the toolbox.*

I learned that insurance companies needed to know the diagnosis before they could pay the doctors I was working for while I trained. Medicine, in practice, was all about finding a name for the problem that the patient was experiencing. This is how the doctor toolbox works. Somebody comes in, they tell the doctor their symptoms, they have tests, they may have an exam, and the doctor determines what the diagnosis is. In the traditional Western medicine world, we can't figure out what to do unless we actually name that problem. Then, we can go into our toolbox and find the right tool.

Medications and Surgery

In my toolbox were thousands of medications that I could choose to give patients. At first, it was exciting because, through these medications, I knew I would have the ability to manipulate so many aspects of people's lives. Using prescriptions, I would be able to help them sleep, bring down their blood pressure, bring down their blood sugar, help their digestion, help their depression, and relieve all kinds of other symptoms.

But I quickly realized that what I was doing with these medications was basically putting a bandage on my patient. Every time my patient came in, I was providing them with a diagnosis and a medication. The medication might address their symptoms in some way, but often, I found that it wasn't solving the problem.

What else was in the toolbox?

Besides the medications, the toolbox contained referrals for surgery and very little else. I realized, over time, that this was what Western medicine was all about. It was the finding of a diagnosis followed by digging in the toolbox to figure out either what medication I should give to help manipulate the problem—put a bandage on it—or where I should send this person to get their problem fixed using surgery or some other physical modality.

I was *so* frustrated! I would watch people come back in within months with more complaints and furthering of their troubles.

And what did I have to give them?

Lots of compassion, and *more drugs.*

I realized only a couple of years into practice that this was not what I signed up for when I decided to go into medicine.

I had dreamed of being a doctor and now that I was, I couldn't even help my patients.

Not only that, but with every passing year, we were seeing chronic diseases, like diabetes, obesity, heart disease, cancer, and autoimmune disease, increase in epidemic proportions. We were also seeing great increases in general complaints like fatigue, sleep issues, foggy brain, pain, gut issues, mood issues, and weight gain.

What is happening to our population? I wondered. *Is there a way to prevent all this misery from happening in the first place?*

More and more medications were being developed and this was the way modern medicine was evolving. It was like a train running out of control.

I knew there had to be a better way.

Only One Tree to Climb

Our human body is so complex, and there are so many things going on at the same time—on a biochemical level, a cellular level, and a physiological level. There are many perspectives we can take when studying the body and its functions. What I have realized over time is that we in Western medicine, although we save many lives, have only learned to bark up one tree. That tree has only two branches of treatment: drugs and surgery.

Western medicine, although well established, is relatively new in the history of medicine—it's just a few hundred years old. My father was a physician, and he was a book collector. When I went through his book collection a few years ago, I found a very old *Physician's Desk Reference,* which is a large book that lists every medication that doctors could use in the year of publication. The version I found was dated 1872, and when I looked in it, I was surprised.

Almost every single medicine that was listed in there was an herb, a plant, or a mineral.

I realize how much medicine has changed in the last one hundred and fifty years. Now, doctors put their faith in what the pharmaceutical companies tell them; we don't even look at the natural medicine world. We rely only on medications that have been created in laboratories.

These remedies sometimes cause other problems. For example, somebody who has heartburn might go to a doctor, and the doctor will give that person an antacid, or a medication that reduces acid production, so the heartburn symptoms will go away. The purpose of those medications is to lessen the amount of acid in the stomach so the juices from the stomach don't burn the patient's esophagus. It seems logical. However, there is another consideration.

The esophageal sphincter—the muscular structure between the stomach and the esophagus—is designed to close when the stomach has an appropriately high level of acid in it. When everything is working right, the sphincter closes under high acid conditions so that these juices stay in the stomach and don't travel up the esophagus.

When patients take medications that reduce acid, this can result in the stomach not having enough acid in it to be able to keep the esophageal sphincter closed. Therefore, many people who are on antacids and proton pump inhibitors (PPIs) are getting a treatment that actually makes things worse instead of making things better. Many of these people are reliant on a treatment—which isn't solving their problem—for the rest of their lives. It also decreases their stomach acid so they can't digest the foods they need to digest, and this can cause levels of nutrients to plummet.

Another example of problematic medication can be seen in the case of autoimmune dis-eases.

These illnesses happen because the body, for some reason, is triggered into creating antibodies against itself. If you have an autoimmune condition, your body is literally attacking itself.

Examples of autoimmune illness are:

- Lupus
- Hashimoto's thyroiditis

- Multiple sclerosis
- Rheumatoid arthritis
- Crohn's disease

With the prevalence of autoimmune disorders on the rise in epidemic numbers, you would think our medical model would be working hard at finding out why.

Right?

Well, we are getting very good at producing medications that suppress the immune system to try to put progression of the disease on hold.

There are more than 140 known autoimmune disorders. There are probably many more. As of sixty to a hundred years ago, many of these disorders hadn't even been described.

The treatments our Western doctors typically offer are strong and dangerous medications that suppress the functioning of your immune system. There are many side effects, and, in addition, depression of the immune system makes people vulnerable to developing other infections and, sometimes, cancer.

In my opinion, these are examples—and you will read many others in this book—of Western medicine barking up the wrong tree.

Are there other trees?

Certainly, there are. Modern Western medicine has climbed so high up in this tree that uses only medications and surgery that they have forgotten to look at the other trees in the forest. There are alternatives that better support the many intertwined activities that are happening in our bodies.

WHAT'S REALLY HAPPENING

Our bodies are fascinating and so complex. The Western medicine tree in the forest has our doctors only focusing on how to beat down the symptoms that patients present, in order to normalize the lab tests that we perform. In standard Western medicine, we have ceased to look at the deeper levels in our bodies. In this section, we will take a brief look at what's happening on these deeper levels.

So Much at the Cellular Level

Let's look at what's going on in our cells. We have so many billions of cells in our bodies. We are made up of all those cells put together. They work together to accomplish all life activities.

What happens inside each of those cells is fascinating. The mitochondria, which are the powerhouses of the cell, are responsible for taking *matter*—our food—and turning it into *energy*, which is how we are able to get out of bed in the morning. There are specialized cells that work together to control communication, digestion, movement, immunity, repair, and reproduction.

Our cells are working constantly and are continually coordinating with each other. There is so much going on at the cellular level in our bodies.

Here are just a few of the cells' activities:

- Making hormones
- Digesting and storing nutrients
- Getting rid of waste products
- Defending against disease-causing microbes
- Making mood chemicals
- Constantly dealing with toxins that come into our bodies
- Repairing and replacing themselves
- Making the chemicals that our cells can use to communicate with each other

The Body on a Larger Level

On a larger level, all parts of our body are interconnected as well. Each organ and each system of our body works with the other organs and systems. When we make a diagnosis, if we look at the body in this interconnected way, we can get a more complete view of the patient. This can help us to treat the patient more effectively.

For example, imagine a patient with pain in his knee. We could examine the patient with a focus on naming the ailment, and simply make a diagnosis—say, arthritis of the knee—and go no further. We would be getting an incomplete picture because what is really going on is a complex series of events and conditions that are culminating in the person experiencing pain in that knee. When we look at the human body, rather than looking at it as its individual parts and individual diagnoses, we need to look at the body as a whole.

This requires asking questions like:

- How good is the communication among all our different organ systems?

- How well is our body using the proteins, carbohydrates, and fats we are taking in?

- How is our nervous system working?

- What is happening with the communication between our cells and our brain with the rest of our body?

- How are our hormones—from adrenal glands, thyroid glands, ovaries, testes—functioning?

- How are these hormones interrelating with everything else in our bodies?

- How well is our gut able to break down the food that we are taking in?

- How well is our gut and immune system functioning to keep the good stuff in and the bad stuff out so that our bodies can work at an optimal level?

Connecting Our Minds and Our Bodies

Another thing that is so important but often overlooked is the relationship between what is going on in our minds and what is going on in our bodies. Many of us don't think enough about this mind-body connection. What's happening in your mind has so much to do with how your body functions.

For example, all the factors below will affect how your body works:

- Your thinking
- Your emotions
- Your mindset
- How you react to stress in your life
- How you relate to people in the world
- Whether you have connections with community
- What you are thinking and feeling as you are waking up in the morning
- What you are thinking and feeling as you are moving through your day

What is going on in our minds has so much to do with how our bodies function.

There are several studies[2] that show one of the biggest common factors—in people who have reached one hundred years old and older— is they have a sense of community, belonging, and relationships.

The science of the relationship between mind and body is very complicated. Our emotions and our mindset can trigger many chemicals. Our mood chemicals, which include neurotransmitters, as well as many of our hormones, are regulated by these thinking processes and emotional processes. When there is more stress, these systems can become overtaxed and imbalanced, affecting what goes on at a cellular level. That can affect our physiology.

It can affect your digestion and determine whether you gain weight. It can affect whether you can lose weight when you want to lose it. It affects what your energy level is and can maybe even impact your sex drive.

Our bodies are just fascinating, and they are so incredibly complex on every level. This complexity may lead you to believe that you have no control over how your body functions, but this isn't so. There may be some things about how your body works that you do not have any control over, but they are few.

---

2 Dan Buettner. *The Blue Zones: Nine Lessons for Living Longer from People Who've Lived the Longest.* National Geographic, 2008.

Patients tell me that they *got diabetes because it runs in the family.* I would hear the same about heart disease, obesity, even fatigue.

There is much more to the story than this.

The truth is that we may be born with a genetic code that could increase our risk for these problems; however, whether or not these problems actually develop is very heavily controlled by how we choose to live, how we eat, and how we take care of ourselves. Ultimately, the progression, or prevention, of most chronic illness is up to us. We are given only one body in this lifetime, and we do have control over how we treat our bodies. The way we treat ourselves impacts how our bodies function.

We can easily forget that we are given only one body in this life, and we may not fully appreciate that our body is the one vehicle through which we can see, feel, and experience our inner and outer world. We have many, many chances to take care of it. Every moment of every day, we have an opportunity to choose to take care of this vehicle. Every moment of every day, it's our choice.

Ready to Work and Play Again

Ethan, thirty-four, was a father of three with one on the way when he came to see us. He had been diagnosed just two years before with ulcerative colitis, an autoimmune disorder of the intestine. He was on heavy doses of immunosuppressant medications and steroids. Worse than that, he never knew when he was going to have an accident. This kept him home a lot and prevented him from playing with his kids. He had to quit his job because of the unpredictability of his gut.

Whenever he did leave his house, he needed to carry a pouch with a change of clothes, just in case. He had asked his gastroenterologist if there were any food changes that might help, and his gastroenterologist said no. He couldn't see himself being so restricted for the rest of his life.

After two months in our program, Ethan still carried his pouch, but it was only to hold his notebook, as he no longer needed a change of clothes. His gut had pretty much normalized, and he hopes to be completely off of his medications in a year. He feels confident with his activities, and he reports that his whole family has adopted his healthy eating habits!

TURNING YOUR HEALTH AROUND

I have had hundreds of patients come into my office and tell me that they are tired and not sleeping; they have gained weight they can't lose; they just don't feel like themselves; or their brains aren't working as well as they used to. Many of them have had tests, and all their tests look normal. Some of them have been told that their complaints are a normal part of aging. When they come in to see me, many tell me they have been told there is nothing they can do about how they are feeling.

I am here to tell you that in most cases, this is completely not true. In most cases, our chronic problems can be turned around. Alongside traditional Western medicine—which is less than two hundred years old—there are many healing traditions, going back to ancient times. Our planet is abundant with fruits, vegetables, nuts, seeds, animals, minerals, and medicinal plants. For thousands of years, cultures have been studying the healing of our bodies using what we have been gifted to live with on this planet.

People had been studying and practicing healing for thousands of years before Western medicine came along. Modern Western medicine has its value, as it has found expertise in helping us bring our bodies back in times of crisis. But much more is available to us, and we should be paying close attention.

We need to tap into all of the wisdom that exists pertaining to healing the human body.

We need to look from all angles, to dig deep into what is going on at a deep level, to sort through all the information, and to act wisely to help our bodies heal from within. Getting down to the root cause of what is happening can allow us to start our healing.

There are many scientists and doctors who, over the past hundred years, have been continuing to research the biochemistry, cell biology and immunology, and other science to help us get to the root cause of our health issues.

Bad Foods Out, Good Nutrition In

It sounds cliché, but we are what we eat. We are what we choose to take into our bodies. In our American culture, advertising and big corporations have helped us to normalize the sale and consumption of food products that are completely unlike what our bodies have been taking in for most of the last several hundred thousand years.

What Americans are eating today has made us part of a huge experiment—an experiment that is answering the question: *What can the human body actually put up with?*

What you take into your bodies is what your body will have to use to perform all the wonderful, complex tasks that it is responsible for day by day. If you don't have the proper nutrition—and, on top of that, if you are taking in lots of toxins—your body cannot function the way it should.

On the other hand, if you bring in the right foods and the right nutrients and you keep out all the things that are challenging your cells and your systems, your body will function so much better.

When you are not sleeping, when you are fatigued, or when you can't lose the weight that you have gained no matter what you do, these are indications that there is an imbalance inside you. It is not normal, and it can be fixed. We can dig down until we find what that imbalance is and turn it around.

Cleaning House—Toxins and Inflammation

Many of the unwanted physical issues that we have in our bodies boil down to inflammation, which we will discuss in more detail in a later chapter. Inflammation happens when our bodies' systems are trying to deal with things that are bothering them.

We are learning more and more about how important our gut is. Our gut not only breaks down our food and digests it, but our gut is responsible for making sure that all the bad stuff we ingest—the dyes, chemicals preservatives, additives, pesticides—stay out of our system and that all the good nutrients get in. We also have a gorgeous balance of good bacteria and other flora in our gut that helps us to digest our food and keeps us healthy.

The system is intricate and requires a healthy balance in order to work well. If your gut system is barraged by chemicals and toxins that are challenging it, it becomes inflamed. When your gut is inflamed, all kinds of things can go wrong. It can leak and let toxins in that don't belong. Inflammation around your gut can cause bloating and belly fat and all kinds of digestive problems.

Most of our immune system is centered in and around our gut, and many of our neurotransmitters and mood chemicals come from our gut. If the gut is not healthy and in balance, this imbalance can result in many of the complaints that we go to our doctors with—fatigue, weight gain, poor sleep, lack of energy, and foggy brain or memory issues.

We have a number of filters in our bodies. Your liver acts as a filter to remove toxins and remove chemicals after you have used them. Your intestine also has a system of detoxification. We have many different systems of detoxification in our bodies. When they are clogged up, just like air filters in your house or your car, they can't work properly.

When we can't detoxify all these chemicals that we are exposed to in our food, air, and environment, then we put even more of a strain on our bodies. By cleaning up that whole system and allowing our filters to work again, we have a great opportunity to help our bodies heal themselves.

Conscious, Proactive Choices Every Day

We have all grown up with our own idea of medicine, which, for most of us, has been affected by the portrayals of the television doctors we grew up watching. We envision a *Marcus Welby* kind of medicine. When we have a problem, we go to the doctor, and the doctor fixes it. The current generation of doctors has grown up with the same idea.

Our whole medical system, with all our medications, tools, and the medication-surgery-toolbox is based on this thought: *We go to the doctor and get fixed.*

If we look back at aboriginal and natural medicine that has been practiced around the world for the past thousands of years, we will find a different approach and a different truth. The truth is that *we* have the most control over how our bodies function—not the doctor.

Many brilliant scientists who are currently studying what is going on at the root of all our functions and health issues in our bodies agree. We have more control over the health of our bodies than what is demonstrated in that model of Western medicine.

Our doctors have a huge role and do many incredible things for us, but it is our responsibility, when it really boils down to it, to look at what is going on in our bodies and what really needs to be fixed.

The onus is on us to take control and be proactive about our bodies. Nobody else is going to do it. Our doctor is not going to do it for us. People who own gyms are not going to do it for us. Even our acupuncturists, our massage therapists, and our homeopaths are not going to do it for us.

They can help you; they can guide you, but the only one who can truly help you is *you*.

Adopting this approach requires us to be proactive about our health. It requires us to look outside the box. It requires us to study, to ask questions, and take action. We must be proactive if we want to turn our health issues around. I can tell you from my experience with hundreds of my patients that it is true that if there is a will, there is a way. Most health care conditions can be turned around if you take the responsibility to make it happen.

This body is your only body, and it is your choice. Be proactive.

When I say that you need to take responsibility for your own health, I don't mean that you need to do it alone. You can seek experts who can guide you. Look for experts who will look at what is going on in your whole body, at all levels.

Look for experts who will try to answer these kinds of questions:

- What is going on at the minute, molecular, microscopic level?

- What is going on at the cellular level?

- What is going on with your body's nutrition, detoxification, toxin loads, digestion, nervous system, and communication?

- What is the relationship between what is happening in your body and what is happening in your mind?

Autoimmune Issues: Finding the Root Cause

Amber was thirty-two years old, working as a make-up artist in Hollywood. She had moved back to our local area to live with her parents, having quit her job because she couldn't do it anymore. She was so extremely fatigued. She also had been gaining a lot of weight and despite spending two hours in the gym six days a week, was unable to lose any weight. She just couldn't function anymore. She had been to multiple doctors who told her that nothing was wrong with her. We did a deeper level of labs and found a number of things going on with her. Her most pressing issue was *Hashimoto's thyroiditis*. This autoimmune disease of the thyroid is becoming more and more common but is often missed by doctors.

The thyroid is one of the most sensitive glands in our bodies to various stressors, including food sensitivities, toxins, sleep issues, and emotional stress. Each of these stressors can cause inflammation in the body which can lead to autoimmune illness. There are over 140 identified autoimmune illnesses, and people who have been diagnosed with one of them are likely to develop others.

By identifying the underlying causes of her autoimmune thyroid, we were able to help her turn her health around. She found multiple sensitivities to foods which were causing gut dysfunction and brain fog. Also, stress from overwork, lack of sleep, poor food choices, and general stress in her job played big roles in the onset of her condition.

She learned new habits. She learned that she needed to take care of her body in order for it to function optimally. She is doing great and back on the film scene in both Los Angeles and Hawaii. And she says that, as long as she takes care of herself and makes the right food choices, she is doing well with good energy and healthy weight.

Testimonials

As a consumer, I felt overwhelmed by choices in health food stores, supplements, and information available. I feel like I've just finished a college course in diet, fitness, and nutrition. It's been incredible to learn so much and now be an informed consumer. I lost twenty pounds. I feel better. I used to write off those little aches and pains to aging but now I can recognize inflammation. I can now make really informed decisions and now it is all about choices.

~ Karyn Shirbroun, 51, Financial Analyst

My PC was stuck in her routine of prescribing new medications for the symptoms I was having. Within three months, I was able to get off diabetic medication, my gut issues are gone, and the brain fog I was experiencing has improved. Now my A1C is below pre-diabetes range. I love the straight-forward curriculum.

~ Martha, 74

I am now a former diabetic.

~ Jonathan Dunn, 75

CHAPTER THREE

What Makes Us Sick

Our bodies are so wonderfully complex. There is so much going on at any given time, but we are conscious about very little. Our bodies do so much behind the scenes—on the larger level, smaller level, and all the levels in between. The more you learn about the human body, the more fascinating it will become.

The cool thing about the body is that everything is interconnected, and everything works together; that also means everything that happens affects everything else. When one function of the body is imbalanced, that can imbalance the rest of the body. In this chapter, we will explore how some of those imbalances and dysfunctions can occur.

HORMONAL IMBALANCES

One of the great regulators in your body is your hormonal system. It is extensive, complicated, and immensely important. You have more than forty hormones, and they are responsible for many diverse activities in your body. They help you to grow and reproduce, they help you to repair, and they keep you functioning efficiently. Each hormone affects different processes, and, in addition, each hormone affects how other hormones are working.

When those hormones are not working in good balance with each other, you can start to experience major problems. Without your hormones in balance, many of the functions in your body that help you to stay healthy and vital will not be able to occur.

We also need to see hormones for the communications network they are in our bodies. Along with neurotransmitters or brain chemicals, these substances are key to the communication between our organs and our cells and are vital for our bodies to be able to function properly, with all parts in sync.

All the hormones are vitally important. Insulin, pregnenolone, melatonin, and other hormones play large roles, but for the purposes of explaining why many people get sick, I am going to concentrate on three: the thyroid hormones, the adrenal hormones, and the sex hormones.

Thyroid

The thyroid gland is one of the major regulators of the functions of your body. In fact, without the thyroid, you wouldn't be able to live at all. The thyroid hormone affects every single cell in your body.

Low thyroid—meaning low levels of thyroid hormones—is one of the most common issues that affect the walking wounded. The thyroid gland is one of the first body parts that responds to any imbalances that the body experiences, including stress, toxins, infections, and imbalances in other organs.

Think about your body as a car, with the thyroid as controlling the gas pedal. When the gas pedal is sluggish, the car—your body—is slow and sluggish. When the thyroid isn't active enough, all the different functions of your body slow down.

Many of the symptoms of low thyroid are just what you might expect from this slowdown:

- Fatigue
- Slower digestion, which causes constipation and other digestive symptoms
- Foggy thinking, or not being able to process things quite as quickly
- Thinning hair and hair loss
- Brittle nails
- Dry skin
- For some people, nerve pain and other aches and pains

Western doctors, from my point of view, often look at the thyroid in a rather cursory manner. The standard screening tests for the thyroid only look at the surface of what is going on. In order to look at the thyroid thoroughly, we need to dig deep. We need to get a series of measurements of several different aspects of the thyroid and get a detailed account of how our patient feels. Even with all the great testing that is available, properly evaluating the symptoms of thyroid deficiency can be the key to getting the thyroid working right.

Thyroid problems have become epidemic in this country. Many people are walking around with thyroid imbalances and have no idea. Someone with thyroid symptoms may consult a doctor, get tested, and be told that they are normal. Getting properly diagnosed is imperative—without correction of a thyroid imbalance, your body can't function properly.

Adrenals

If the thyroid is the gas pedal of our car, then the adrenals are the engine and the ignition switch. Without the adrenals, nothing happens; if you had no adrenal hormones, you wouldn't be alive. Your adrenals are small glands that sit right on top of your kidneys. The adrenal glands make several different hormones, each of which is quite important. The hormone that I will be talking about in this chapter is necessary to your overall health, and it is common to find it out of balance in the walking wounded. That hormone is cortisol.

Cortisol has been dubbed by some as *the twenty-first century stress hormone*.[3] That is because cortisol is produced by our adrenal glands in response to stress.

We have so many stressors in our world. Those stressors can be physical stress like injuries, car accidents, or surgeries. Stressors can also be chemical such as the toxins in our environment and in the foods that we eat regularly.

When we think of stress, most of us think about emotional stress, that feeling of conflict—in relationships, at home, or at work. It is what happens to us when we try to multi-task too much, burning the candle at both ends, not getting enough sleep.

Any time you are stressed, these stressors, in effect, are asking your body for help. The help comes in the form of cortisol from your adrenal glands. You can think of cortisol as helping your motor to accommodate those increased or additional needs.

The difficulty comes when you have lots of stressors in your life or you have long-term stressors. In these cases, your adrenal glands are constantly putting out cortisol, and over time, they can burn out. I see highly stressed patients who come to me complaining of fatigue, with bodies that are just not functioning properly. They typically complain that they

---

3 Wilson, James. *Adrenal Fatigue: The 21ˢᵗ Century Stress Hormone.* Smart Publications, 2001.

have a foggy brain and no "get up and go". They may also be somewhat overweight and tell me they have been trying, but failing, to lose weight.

When I investigate—an investigation that includes a detailed history and specific tests—I find that the adrenal glands in these patients are underperforming. They have just been pooped out from overuse, and as a result, they are not able to produce much adrenal hormone at all.

The good news is that the adrenal glands can heal. It takes special testing to assess the status of the glands, as well as special treatments to help adrenal glands get back into balance. Identifying stressors and working on how stress affects your body is another key to healing your adrenal glands. The walking-wounded patients who have adrenal issues may not have a chance at feeling better without these treatments.

Sex Hormones: Menopause and Manopause

In our bodies, we have lots of other hormones that regulate processes and how we feel. The hormones that come from our ovaries and testes are vitally important in growth and development but are also necessary for the continued maintenance and vitality of many of the systems in our bodies.

Women usually go through menopause sometime in their fifties. At this time, their ovaries, sometimes abruptly, stop producing estrogen, progesterone, and testosterone—yes, women, we *do* make testosterone and it is very important. Men also go through a process of what some people refer to as *andropause,* or *manopause,* during which there is a lowering of testosterone. It happens more gradually than the menopause of women but is also a natural process that occurs with aging.

These sex hormones affect so many aspects of our vitality, including:

- Heart health
- Brain health
- Bone health
- Skin health
- Muscle versus fat ratios
- Energy levels
- Feelings of well-being
- Mood

When your levels of these hormones are low, you can expect that you will experience changes in some of these areas.

Modern medicine has done a good job in the last one hundred years of being able to keep us alive longer. Our life expectancy has increased because of better sanitation, antibiotics, emergency surgery, clean water, and other advances. This brings us to an unprecedented place in history, where we are living longer than we ever have.

About two hundred years ago, humans would live only into their fifties, or maybe into their sixties if they were lucky.

Very few humans lived into their seventies, eighties, or nineties. We have become part of a big experiment by living longer. One of the new variables is the loss of sex hormones that occurs late in age.

In the long term, what happens to our bodies without these hormones?

We are seeing a big growth in memory care centers, nursing homes, and assisted living facilities because people who are living these longer years are becoming extremely fragile, losing their memories, losing their brain power, and having heart attacks and strokes. They essentially have bodies that are still living but are severely disabled. Some of these changes are in part, due to the loss of sex hormones after menopause and andropause.

What would the world look like if we were able to continue maintaining these incredible hormones of vitality?

You are probably aware that synthetic hormones have been developed for medical use. Synthetic hormones are made in the laboratory and marketed by pharmaceutical companies. Bioidentical hormones, while made in a laboratory, are identical to the molecules that our bodies naturally make. There is a big difference.

In 2001 and 2002, two large studies were published that concluded that the synthetic hormones, Premarin and Provera, when used for Hormone Replacement Therapy

(HRT) in menopausal women, increased these women's risk of breast cancer and heart disease. At that time, many, many women who had been relying on HRT to help with symptoms of menopause or for help in preventing or treating degenerative conditions associated with loss of hormones— such as osteoporosis, changes to vaginal wall leading to painful intercourse, or depression—were abruptly taken off these medications. As you can imagine, or may have experienced, there were a lot of unhappy women and frustrated physicians.

The good news is that hundreds of studies have been done so far on the use of bioidentical hormones. In contrast to the studies on the synthetic hormones, bioidentical hormones appear to show a high level of safety and do not show any increased risk for heart disease or cancer. In fact, the bulk of literature suggests that they are protective against the occurrence of these issues.[4] I am happy to say that for most people, bioidentical hormones appear to be quite safe and only a good thing.

Are hormone supplements right for you?

When I work with patients whose bodies may be affected by a loss or imbalance of hormones, we have an in-depth discussion about options. Making this choice is a very personal thing, so I work closely with each of my patients to evaluate whether hormone replacement is right for them.

---

4 Rouzier, Neal. *How to Achieve Healthy Aging.* Wordlink Medical Publishing, 2012.

First, it is very important to address and correct underlying issues that may be at the roots of these imbalances. And, we may find that either temporarily or permanently, using bioidentical hormones to balance a woman's system can change her world.

Can women of childbearing age also have sex hormone issues?

Absolutely, and it is common. As a result of our lifetime exposures to toxins, our body's response to sugar and carbohydrates, and sometimes imbalances in other glands like our thyroid or adrenals, many women can find themselves with an imbalance in their sex hormones. This can cause all kinds of problems, like premenstrual symptoms, heavy periods, headaches, weight gain, acne, male-pattern hair growth, and mood issues. Getting to the root cause of these hormone imbalances and correcting them can be the difference between misery and happiness. I have seen it thousands of times.

I have only touched the surface regarding these great communicators—the hormones. Besides the ones I mentioned here, there are many others that play important roles. Hormones give us vitality and play a crucial role in the communication between body systems. They are necessary to all aspects of our body function, making them one of the most critical areas that we evaluate and treat in root cause medicine.

INFLAMMATION

Inflammation is a body response that influences almost every body function and so, results in a wide variety of symptoms.

Why does inflammation happen?

I like to think of inflammation as our body's way of dealing with things that it either isn't sure about or that it doesn't like. Most inflammation results from the natural functioning of the immune system. We will discuss this in more detail below.

What Is Inflammation and What Causes It?

Our immune systems are made up of many different kinds of cells that have different ways of dealing with intruders into the body. Those intruders can be toxins, or other substances that our bodies don't like or don't know what to do with. Sometimes they can be pathogens, such as viruses or bacteria; and sometimes they can be food-like substances that our bodies just can't recognize.

Did you know that, since World War II, 70,000–80,000 new toxins have been released into the United States?

Toxins can come in the forms of pesticides, herbicides, dyes, preservatives, and heavy metals. We are exposed to them every day.

What happens when your body comes into contact with something that it doesn't recognize?

The cells of the immune system activate in response to the encounter. Different cells will have different strategies to deal with intruders. Some can create chemicals or release antibodies; some attack pathogens or destroy toxins. The immune system is like a whole military system that has been created to isolate, surround, and destroy the substances that our bodies can't use.

When the immune system gets activated, lots of these immune cells accumulate either in a specific area of the body, or if the toxins are everywhere, then all over the body. Once immune cells are activated, chemicals designed to set the stage for attacking the unfamiliar substance and repairing any damage it has caused are released. One of the side effects is an accumulation of fluid—what we call *swelling*.

This accumulation of fluid and cells can be local, such as you see around a cut, or it can be more generalized.

Interestingly, over 70 percent of our immune system is housed in and around our gut. And, because so many of the intruders or toxins come through our gastrointestinal system, this means that lots of inflammation can happen.

If the inflammation happens around our gut, we might see a bloating or swelling around the belly, which might look or feel like belly fat. The inflammation can become more generalized or travel to all parts of our body and that can cause big issues like foggy brain, fatigue, sleep issues, headaches, loss of stamina, or pain.

Inflammation is a necessary part of life and helps us heal from cuts and wounds in surgeries, so it is quite important and necessary for us to live. Many people who are suffering from illnesses and are not feeling well may find that inflammation is a major cause of their symptoms.

Symptoms of Inflammation

Inflammation can look different in different patients. If you have a cut or a bee sting, inflammation might look like a little bit of swelling of the skin. There might be some redness. However, inflammation can be invisible to the human eye, even to the doctor, when it is happening deep inside the body.

One of the most common areas where inflammation may occur is in or around the gut. Your gut is responsible for taking nutrients in, but it is also responsible for keeping bad things out. It houses more than 70 percent of your immune system. When the bad things do come around, your gut area produces inflammation to deal with the bad stuff and send it out of our bodies. From the gut, this inflammation can travel around our bodies and wreak havoc on virtually everything.

The symptoms of inflammation are many and varied.

For example:

- Joint and muscle inflammation can cause pain and stiffness.

- It can increase the swelling that already exists in arthritic joints, which increase symptoms of arthritis.

- It can be a major cause of brain fog and memory issues.

- It can result in low stamina or fatigue.

- It can cause many gut symptoms, including gas, bloating, diarrhea, or constipation.

- It can cause weight gain and belly fat as the defenses of the immune system sequester toxins and store them in fat cells, signaling a toxic overload. Weight gain and belly fat can therefore be signs of a toxic overload in your body.

Why Is It So Important?

When inflammation is causing symptoms, like some of those I just mentioned, how is it affecting the biochemical and physiological processes in our bodies?

It has a wide range of effects. Inflammation can lead to major hormone dysfunction. It can lead to problems with our sugar and insulin system, which can lead to pre-diabetes, diabetes, weight issues, and belly fat. That is a process called *insulin resistance*.

Scientists are now studying inflammation and its impact on cardiovascular problems, including atherosclerosis—hardening of the arteries—and clot formation that can lead to stroke and heart attacks. Cholesterol is not the only problem in this area; in fact, it is likely that inflammation might even be more important than cholesterol as a factor in cardiovascular disease.

Inflammation is felt to be a major cause of Alzheimer's disease and other brain disorders. Scientists are studying the relationship between inflammation and brain conditions like Attention Deficit Disorder/Attention Deficit Hyperactivity Disorder (ADD/ADHD), autism, Parkinson's disease, multiple sclerosis, and even mood disorders such as depression or anxiety. Removing inflammation is one of the first things that we start working on when we see our patients who are having any of these issues.

Inflammation can dramatically affect the functioning of our bodies. Paying attention to inflammation and reducing the causes and effects of the inflammation are key to improving health and vitality.

A Fuller Life With Better Health

Debbie D. is sixty-eight years old and works as a state government employee. Debbie came to me because she was at the end of her rope. She had been suffering since the age of fourteen with chronic diarrhea that had gotten so bad that she was no longer leaving her house even to take walks because she was afraid that she wouldn't make it back to her bathroom in time. She had completely given up all of her social activities.

Other symptoms included a longstanding history of *fibromyalgia* with chronic pain. She also was complaining of a foggy brain, hair loss, chronic asthma, and her abdominal issues, which also included frequent discomfort and cramping in her gut. Debbie started on a program with us that helped her to remove from her diet the foods that were harming her, to repair her gut, and rebalance it.

Within two months, most of her symptoms had turned around. She had a completely normal bowel pattern and she had completely normal bowel movements. She was no longer concerned at all about incontinence. She started leaving her house and becoming very active in her community. She no longer needed her inhalers for asthma, her hair stopped falling out and had become thicker again, and her clarity of mind came back to a point where she felt very sharp. When I saw her after eight weeks, she was extremely active and making plans for the future. One year later, she has bought a vacation cabin, is in a long-term relationship, and is making plans to do all the things that she had always wanted to do but had be unable to do because of her health.

MATTER AND ENERGY

One of the most common complaints that my patients come to me with is fatigue. Low energy can affect every second, minute, and hour of a person's day. Fatigue certainly affects the choices you make, and it can dramatically impact the quality of your life. Your energy level will determine how much you are going to be able to do in your day, as well as the kinds of things you are going to be able to do.

Energy is vitally important to the functioning of our one and only body. Here are some more thoughts on energy issues in the body.

What Is Our *ON* Button?

Functionally, it all boils down to the fact that our bodies run on the energy that is made from matter. We take in food in the form of many different kinds of nutrients as well as carbohydrates, proteins, and fats. The diverse and complex systems in our bodies take that matter and convert it into energy for our life activities. This conversion is a chemical process that happens in our cells.

Where is the *ON* button for this conversion of food into energy?

As we already discussed, much of this complex process occurs in tiny little parts in each of our cells called the *mitochondria*. It is here where, through a complex number of functions, we are turning our nutrients into energy.

Because of the complexity of this process, there are many things that can go wrong. Because our cells need a regular supply of energy to continue to function, we need to safeguard the cellular activities that provide energy.

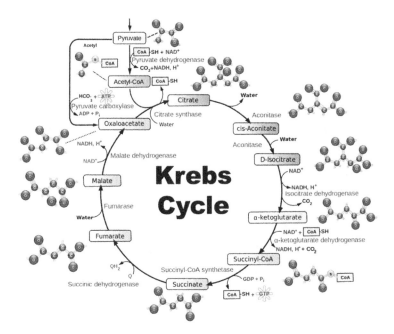

How can we best support this process?

Supporting Energy Production

To make this process efficient, we need to provide a healthy environment for our cells, especially elements that affect:

- Mitochondrial health
- The supply of nutrients
- The supply of oxygen
- The clearing out of waste products

The mitochondria are the powerhouses where most of our usable energy supply is produced. We need a steady supply

81

of good nutrients for these processes, and oxygen is required as well. In addition, it is important for powerhouse efficiency that our bodies are able to clean out anything that they don't need, including toxins and metabolic waste products.

Several elements can compromise this system. As I said earlier, lack of supplies or an unhealthy environment for the mitochondria can cause inefficiency and fatigue. One item we may not give much consideration in this area is the importance of sleep. In addition to giving us rest, there are certain functions that happen during sleep that are of utmost importance in keeping our systems running.

These include:

- Much of our detoxification
- Cell repair
- Cell growth
- The making of hormones
- The making of neurotransmitters—brain chemicals that are responsible for our emotions
- The processing speed and ability of the brain

Under ideal circumstances, a complete revitalization happens during our sleep, in addition to the processing of many of the emotions and experiences that we have had during the prior day. If our sleep is not long or deep enough, these processes can't happen. That can cause many problems.

Another vital issue is oxygen. In order to access the wonderful energy found in our foods, adequate levels of oxygen must be regularly supplied. There are many different ways that this supply can be jeopardized. People who suffer sleep apnea may not know it, but their oxygenation—the amount of oxygen they get during the night—may get to dangerously low levels. In addition, many of us have a habit of holding our breath all day and don't do enough deep breathing to get good oxygen to our tissues. Also, if you smoke or take certain pain, calming, or sleep medications, you may also be compromising your body's capacity to get oxygen to your tissues.

The supply of proper nutrients is essential for energy production. As I have said several times, if we don't have the nutrients we need, we can't support the processes that we need to keep our bodies functioning.

Sugar plays a vital role in the energy fluctuations of your body. When you eat, your sugar rises, and it causes the release of a hormone called insulin, which will then take the sugar out of the bloodstream. This is a necessary and vital process to keep you alive. However, if you eat lots of sugar or eat meals heavy in carbohydrates several times during the day, you cause repeated fluctuations in your levels of blood sugar throughout the day. Repeated fluctuations in blood sugar can lead to periods of blood sugar getting low. Blood sugar is vital to the functioning of your brain and the rest of your body. When your blood sugar decreases, that can cause a major crash in your energy.

Your body can make fuel only from what it has. Sleep, oxygenation, nutrients, and proper regulation of blood sugar are all vitally important and directly connected to our levels of energy.

Why Do We Get Tired?

When we are thinking about energy, we need to pay attention to what is happening all over the body. When fatigue is a symptom, many factors need to be evaluated and addressed. The whole picture matters because everything affects everything else. The body is a complex network. There are so many different functions and interconnected systems.

I have spoken about some different factors that can cause us to be tired, but here is a more complete list:

- Hormone imbalances
- Blood sugar fluctuations
- Poor or inadequate sleep
- Stress
- Mood issues like depression or anxiety
- Inflammation or toxic load
- An underlying viral, bacterial, or other infection

Dis-ease is a complicated thing. Our bodies are intricate, incredible, and extremely complicated. What makes us not feel well or what underlies a disease process can be complicated to sort out. However, with the proper practitioner who addresses problems in an organized and straightforward manner, you can get to the bottom of what is causing you to be having the health issues that you are having and figure out what needs to be done to turn them around.

Testimonials

I've lost weight. Most importantly is how I look and feel. I can get up early and not crash late in the afternoon. My brain is more clear. I can focus on my volunteer work better. My cholesterol had gotten really high, and I was put on Lipitor. Through this program my cholesterol as well as blood pressure have come way down.

~ Candace Manary, 67

I had pain in my right side. Every time I ate, it got worse. Doctors couldn't find the cause for over a year. I was losing hope it would get better. Now, food is not an enemy anymore. I feel better and have energy. I am back to my normal routine and activities.

~ Candi Baker, 66

Losing weight and inches without having to starve myself or kill myself with a rigorous exercise routine. Loving the food. I feel nourished, *not just full. I'm not starving and ripping into anything I can find in the cupboards. It's such a different feeling. Haven't had a headache (chronic daily headaches) since the first week when I was going off sugar. Yay!*

~ Kari Duron, 40, Mother of Three

CHAPTER FOUR

Turning Your Health Around

THE WHOLE PICTURE

Do you think you are stuck with your long-term health issues?

Many people do. If you are not sleeping well, suffer from fatigue, or if you can't lose weight, you might think that you are stuck with these symptoms. The truth is that most people are *not* stuck with the maladies that they have.

When we go to our doctors, we usually have a distinct set of individual complaints, and Western doctors respond in kind, dealing with each problem individually. What we really need to do is to look at the whole picture.

Western Medicine Versus Root Cause Medicine

Western medicine is so good at so many things. It is so good at keeping us alive when we are far down the path of our illness. When it comes to our everyday symptoms and chronic illnesses that keep getting worse, however, we should be looking at the body in a much more comprehensive way.

As I have said, the Western medical doctors typically regard health and disease in a very specific way. This is apparent when we consider medical specialties. If you have a thyroid issue, you might be sent to an endocrinologist; if you have an autoimmune issue, you may be sent to a rheumatologist; for arthritis symptoms, you might be sent to an orthopedist. Each doctor is expert at diagnosis and prescribing the appropriate medical treatment for conditions within the realm of their training.

Also, as I discussed earlier, medicine has grown over the years to value a toolbox that deals with the symptoms of the current problem—to change lab values or alleviate symptoms—rather than to get to the root cause of the issues. The problem with just treating your symptoms or your lab values is that, despite all the medications you take, your health issues are likely going to continue to get worse and not better.

The truth is, when we look at each of these things, we don't have to look at them separately—we can look at them together. When we look at different conditions or symptoms all together, we can see root causes that are common to many of these different ailments.

When we look at health issues this way, instead of just looking at one disease or another, we are looking at the *whole* person. We are able to see the whole picture and when we do this, we are able to get the healing done from the bottom up and the inside out.

The Right Tests

One of the most important health necessities is to get the right testing done. When we go to our doctors, only basic lab tests are usually ordered. Many of you who have had complaints and have gone to your doctors have been told that your tests are all normal. I call these the *Are You About to Die?* tests. They are extremely important, and they are necessary; however, they don't go nearly deep enough to really give us a picture of what is going on with you. The truth is that there are many other tests available. Using appropriately chosen specialized tests, we have the ability to dig deeper down, to look at the root of what is going on in our bodies. But these tests are often not done.

There are tests that look at your nutrient and vitamin levels or assess how your gut is working. Some tests look at toxins or allergies. Tests can tell you what's going on with your sleep. A focused and meaningful investigation is necessary to figure out what is happening in your body, to find the root causes of symptoms. Without this kind of testing, we as doctors are running blind.

Putting It All Together

In order to be able to look at the big picture, we need to look at all the different components of what is going on in your health. Then we need to put it together. One of my favorite things to do is to sit down with my patients, after having performed an in-depth health history, as well as a family history, and having gotten a comprehensive deep set of labs. I talk with my patients about lifestyle, diet, and health goals, as well as levels of stress and attitudes about health.

When we look at the big picture of a patient's health, we are then able to sit down, put it all together, and see what is really going on in your body. Only then can we really see what is possible. Only then can we take the next step and see the healing happen on a comprehensive basis, from the inside out.

It is so important to be able to look at everything because every single piece matters. Every single piece of who you are—from what's going on physically in your body to how you live your life on a daily basis—plays into how you feel and how your body is working on a daily basis.

GETTING BACK IN BALANCE

Once you look at the big picture with your doctor, you can really see what is going on in your health. Everything will become very clear—what is in balance, what is out of balance, and what direction you need to start moving in to start getting you back into balance.

Those symptoms you have—poor sleep, fatigue, depression, or weight issues—are knocking on your door. Your body is knocking on your door to let you know that something is out of balance. Answer the door, and then you can start the process of getting everything back into balance.

All Systems in Working Order

We have several systems in our bodies that need to work together in order to keep us in great working order. To get things back in balance, we need to take a good look at what is most important.

When someone has health issues, here are some of the most common areas of concern:

- The gut
- Inflammation
- Toxin filtration
- Energy processes
- Body movement

We have already discussed how inflammation can impact our bodies. We also need to consider what kinds of toxins our bodies are dealing with and how the filters in our bodies are able to filter those toxins. We need to assess how efficiently our cells extract energy out of the foods that we eat and what we can do to help enhance that process. In addition, we should consider how our body is moving, as movement is so important to all the different processes that keep us functioning well.

We must evaluate every symptom individually, and then see how they may be working together. Then, we can correct imbalances and get optimum health.

Optimizing Nutrition

The food you eat can either be the safest and most powerful form of medicine or the slowest form of poison.
~ Ann Wigmore
The Hippocrates Diet and Health Program

At the same time you are getting your systems back into balance, you also should be looking at your nutrition. It is true—you actually *are* what you eat.

What is going into your body?

Are you giving your body the nutrients that it needs?

Are you poisoning yourself slowly?

As a traditionally trained doctor, I can say that until the last decade or so, for Western medical doctors, *food as medicine* has been a foreign concept. I remember my father, who was a wonderful and well-respected family doctor between 1951 and 1990, telling me that what we eat does not have a lot to do with how our bodies work. I think that this mid-twentieth century view of food likely came from the fact that because, prior to the mid 1900s, most of our food, by definition, was organic and the soil in which our food was grown *was* full of good nutrients—we didn't need to think about it. Of course, our food supply today is a much different story. Some would argue that the concept of *food as medicine* is still fairly foreign. And, the concept of *food as poison* has been equally as foreign. Some of this lack of concern for the quality of our nutrition may also have come from the influence our food and drug industries have had on our thinking.

Much of what we need can come from our daily food, but sometimes supplementation is necessary. We all need to pay attention in a detailed way to what we are taking in and how our bodies are processing it. Take a good look at what you are exposing yourself to and determine what is not serving you so you can eliminate whatever is unnecessary or unhealthy.

Momentum Moving Forward

It's taken a long time for your body to get to where it is today. You should be aware that just as it takes time to wind things up, it will take time to unwind.

Most of your cells will replace themselves regularly. Some replace themselves within a few days, many will replace themselves within a year, and others may take up to seven years. As the cells change, as your nutrition changes, all the other aspects of how your body is functioning will also be making changes—but these changes can take time.

Transformation takes time. Just as the world wasn't built in a day, we can't turn ourselves around in a day.

Transformation takes commitment. It's important to walk into this process with the attitude that it is going to take time and commitment to turn things around. With all long-term processes and transformations, the big key is mindset and attitude. It also takes time and commitment for us to find out what works for our own bodies individually and what helps us to heal and to function properly.

When you start the process of healing your body from the inside out, it can feel overwhelming at the beginning. Typically, if you persist, you will start to see that the small changes you have made in the way you approach health initiate big changes in your body.

Often, big changes happen pretty quickly—it is not uncommon for someone to experience big changes in their levels of energy, quality of sleep, and brain function in just a few short weeks. Even cravings can turn around quickly when the body gets into balance. For others, the changes can be slower and subtler.

Understanding the process—seeing how what you do will affect your life in the long term—is important. Getting the wheel turning and keeping the momentum can help you self-propel the whole process because once the changes start, you'll want them to continue going that way.

When they're fairly far down the line, many people tell me that the changes they've made have not been so hard. The benefits have been so enormous that they find that the work they've done is work they want to continue, and it's simply become new habit, so it's not as hard as they thought it would be.

It is not that difficult to start getting your body back in balance. It does take time, it does take commitment, and it does take change on your part. I have guided hundreds of people through it; most people had initial concerns about being able to follow through and were delighted that the changes were very straightforward and the results so significant. You were only given one body in this lifetime, and what you do with it is completely your choice. What I am telling you is that it is possible to make big changes and get your body back in balance if that is where you want to go.

Rebalancing

Kristen joined us because she had lost her world due to her illness. At thirty-two, she was simply exhausted. She had given up her physical therapy practice and had become a homebody. She was no longer able to keep a social life, and she was worried about losing her relationship with her husband. She desperately wanted to start a family but could not see embarking on that while feeling the way she did.

Kristen was a beautiful, trim, healthy-appearing young woman, one I would call part of the walking wounded. Nobody would have looked at her and thought she was anything but completely healthy. Her doctors said her screening labs were fine; they wouldn't take a second look at her. A deep-level set of labs revealed that Kristen was suffering from an autoimmune disorder of her thyroid. Because autoimmune disorders are commonly a result of imbalances in the gut, toxic load, food sensitivities, or other issues that cause inflammation and disruption of the immune system, we dug down deep to help her rebalance her system.

Six months later at her final visit, Kristen reported that she had rented a space to start her physical therapy practice again. Even better, she was pregnant!

MAKING CHANGE REAL

Earlier in my Functional Medicine practice, before I adopted my current model, I was finding that my patients were having a hard time getting started or making lasting change. No matter what I did—sitting with them for hours, giving detailed instructions, giving them marching orders, meeting them monthly—many times my patients would come back and say that the change was too hard, or they hit a road block. They might proceed well for a little while, and then something would get in their way and they would fail. Finally,

I decided that I needed to look for a better model of care that would help my patients make change for real and for good.

In my research, I found that the three main components to making real change are:

- Education
- Structure
- Good mentoring

It's not magic, but a combination of education, structure, and mentoring will enable us all to be able to make a change for real. I will discuss each of these components below.

Education

Education is vital.

If we don't know why we are doing something, why would we want to do it?

Why would we be motivated to take on a practice or make a change when we have no idea why we're doing it?

We need to educate ourselves about how our bodies function, but more than this, we need to know this information on a deep level, an experiential level. You need to know how your *own* body functions and what your individual needs are. Knowing that is vital to help you be motivated to make the changes that you need to make and keep them going, to make for lasting health. Think of it as a college course: *Your Own Body*.

For example, knowing how certain foods react in your body is vital to helping you make a decision whether or not you want to eat those foods. For example, if nightshade vegetables make your arthritis worse, or if eating wheat causes you to feel heavy and bloated, this is important information that will help guide your moment-to-moment decisions about how you are going to live your life and treat your body.

If you don't know these things, how are you going to make a change?

Structure

How many times have you decided that you wanted to do something—you wanted to lose weight, you wanted to take guitar lessons, or you wanted to start a creative project—and your feeling about it was so very strong?

You felt so good when you made that decision, but then, when you looked back a month later or two months later, you realized that you didn't actually start that project or didn't actually get that mission accomplished. The primary reason people fail when they have an idea and don't achieve it is they don't have a plan. This is what happens most often. Having a plan, knowing what is happening now, what is happening next, what is happening in the short-term future and long-term future, is vital to being able to stay with a program and to stay on top of what needs to happen to make that change that you need to make.

Mentoring

One of the biggest mistakes that many of us make is to think we can do everything on our own. There are many things that we are capable of doing on our own, but many of them require the help of someone else. The trick is to know the difference.

For me, for example, I know that when it comes to matters of taxes or law, I need to get some help. I need to get help from someone who is an expert in these fields. This may seem obvious, and most people would agree that it makes sense to find help for these kinds of tasks.

When it comes to more subtle things like negotiating health issues, however, many of us think we can do them on our own. The truth is that the most successful people have coaches. The best athletes in the world have coaches. The best coaches in the world have coaches.

None of us would want to get on an airplane with a pilot who has learned to fly a plane just by reading a book or taking online courses. We want that pilot to have sat in an airplane for many hours with somebody by their side helping them learn what they need to learn along the way. We want their technique to be the best it can be.

Yes, there are some things we can do on our own, but when it comes to having success in areas that might be a little bit new to us or complicated or challenging, it's really important that we let ourselves be guided by people who have expertise in the field.

Having a coach leads to a much greater chance of having success, so why not?

Testimonials

After only 3 months I had much less brain fog. I'm sleeping through the night, my stress level is way down, I've got lots of energy and I'm enthusiastic about things.

I'm really glad I came here, and I would recommend it to anyone who is motivated to not feel old when you're not really old!
~ Claudia Dow, 67, Retired Teacher

I was tired of being sick and heavy. I had tried all kinds of diets and plans and never had success, until I came here. I have lost thirty-eight pounds so far am having no trouble keeping it off. I am off blood pressure medications, feeling better, my sense of worth is now high, and my overall outlook is great!
~ David Smith, 56

[I had been] struggling with weight and energy levels for the past ten years. There were times it was a challenge for me, but I stuck with it! I'm now down thirty pounds and my joints hurt less, which is huge. I am sleeping solidly through the night and actually feel rested in the morning.

My last blood tests showed almost all of my numbers in the normal range, where I was borderline diabetic before.

Overall, I think I have given myself the gift of a happy life by doing this program. I highly recommend it.

~ Catherine Welsh, 62, Music Teacher

CHAPTER FIVE

Act and Take Personal Responsibility

ONE BODY IN THIS LIFE

I think no matter what our religion or spirituality, most of us can agree that we are given one body in this life. This body is a tool. It is the only tool of its kind, and we need to use it to make our way through this world all through our unique, particular life.

Body as a Gift and a Tool

You can look at your body as a gift. This gift has been given to make the most of your life in this world, to do whatever you were meant to do. No matter who you are—mother, father, daughter, son, grandparent, friend, community member, entrepreneur, or someone who is here to be of great service to everyone else in their life—your body is your tool. How your body functions directly affects how well you are able to perform in the world and how rewarding your life is for you.

Author Augusten Burroughs wrote, "When you have your health, you have everything. When you do not have your health, nothing else matters at all."[5]

If you are feeling tired, or your brain isn't functioning optimally, or your mood is low, or you feel bad about yourself, it affects you deeply. It affects how you are with your significant other, with your family, and with your friends. It affects how you act when you are out there in the world, and it affects what is important to you.

If you feel badly about the way you look in your clothes, or if you feel poorly, whether it be physically, emotionally, or mentally, these feelings can get in the way of you being who you want to be in the world and what you are able to bring to the world.

Our Choices Drive Our Functions

It's true that the bodies we are born with have a unique genetic code, which gives our bodies the template for how we are going to look and, in some ways, how we are going to function. However, only a small percentage of our genetics is not modifiable, meaning that we have the ability, no matter what genes we are born with, to influence most of the functions of our body.

---

5 Burroughs, Augusten. *Dry: A Memoir*. Macmillan, 2013. 286.

How you live, both in the short term and in the long term, has a huge effect on both the everyday and long-term functions of your body. Every choice that you make in the moment—and you make thousands of choices—influences your body in the long term.

What are your choices like?

For example:

- What do you choose to eat?
- How much sleep do you give yourself?
- What chemicals do you choose to expose your body to?
- How do you respond to stress?
- Do you exercise?
- How do you care for yourself emotionally and spiritually?
- What do you challenge yourself with physically and mentally?

Your choices can make or break how your body functions, how long you live, and what your quality of life looks like in your middle and later years.

What Do You Want to Accomplish in This Life?

Some of you may be fortunate enough to have a very clear vision of why you are living your unique and individual life. Others may not have as clear an understanding.

What's your *why?*

Stop for a moment and think. Search your feelings and you will probably find some answers.

Consider these questions as you are thinking:

- Why are you here?
- What's your purpose?
- Who depends on you?
- Who needs you to be healthy?
- Who needs you to be here for as long as you can?
- Who needs you to be active and independent for as long as you can?
- What do you want to accomplish in this life?
- What's on your bucket list?

I invite you to stop for a moment. Try and figure out your why.

What is it that has made you come this far reading in this book, and why is it that you want to be in the best health that you can be?

Cultivate the kind of vision that comes from being able to answer these questions. It can help to drive you from the inside when you are making your moment-to-moment daily and lifestyle choices.

You are given this one body. You have great control over many aspects of how it works. It is your choice to take care of this one body or not. The choices you make will determine how your body is going to function.

IS THERE EVER A GOOD TIME?

I have had countless people sitting in my office who pay me good money to talk about how dissatisfied they are with their health and how much they want their bodies to be working differently than they are. They talk about how much their issues with their bodies get in the way of their abilities to be fully present in their lives and to accomplish what they want to accomplish.

When I talk to them about the fact that in order to feel better, they are going to need to make some changes—perhaps in their diet or in their lifestyle—they often procrastinate. When I speak about the need to invest a little bit of money to get the lab studies and help that they need, they may have difficulty prioritizing their need for health. They may find it difficult to opt for the changes they need to make for their health in favor of all the other things that are vying for their attention in their lives, like work and vacations, house projects, or the many other ways they want to spend their time, energy, effort, and finances.

When is it the right time to prioritize your health?

The answer is NOW. Although you will always have other important areas to worry about in your life, when you improve your health, it will improve every other area of your life.

Procrastination as Our Comfort Zone

It has taken all of us a long time to develop the habits we have today. We are comfortable with our habits. In fact, we have developed many of them because they are comfortable. However, if these habits are no longer serving you or if they are getting in your way of being able to get your health back, it may be time to take a critical look at what these habits are and how badly you need them.

I am a born procrastinator, so I know full well how difficult it is to make changes. When you make a change, the change needs to come from inside yourself, and it needs to come from that *why* we discussed in the last section—from your inner desire to have things be different than they are.

I think that procrastination itself is a comfort zone for most of us. What I have seen is that when people can move past that toxic train of thought, they can make an enormous difference in how their body functions. It is often a matter of just taking those first baby steps, just to get the cogs of the wheels turning. Soon the new changes are noticeable, and it seems to get easier after that.

No Time Like the Present

Many times, after a consultation with a patient in my office, I have felt very sad. I have spent hours with patients, listening to their woes and concerns and complaints and every detail that is overwhelming them about how their body is no longer working for them. They say they are missing their life and it is passing by them. They also say they are very fearful about the likely progression of their health issues, like heart attack, stroke, or losing their legs or eyes or kidneys; or even they fear that they will spend their next and last twenty years on their couch or in a nursing facility because their bodies won't be able to let them do the things they want to do. They tell me how they want or need their lives to be, but when we talk about taking those first couple of steps and starting to make some change, the walls often go right up. I can tell that they are rejecting the idea, and it makes me sad.

They start to talk about how they are thinking of taking a vacation soon, or have a child's wedding coming up, or the holidays are nearing. They say they are going to be moving soon or they are planning to remodel their house, and they just don't know if they can make the time or set aside the finances to be able to make the changes that are necessary for their health.

Sitting right in front of me, they may have just told me that their issues are completely overwhelming and damaging, and that they can't live with them anymore. However, when the discussion turns to doing something about it, the idea of starting now to fix their problems often seems to be out of the question.

What I have learned over the many years I have been in practice is that the people who succeed in making changes start with baby steps, and they start with them right away. They don't go home to think about it; they don't put it off until next week or next month or next year. They realize that the issues that are going on within are not going to change unless they do start to take those baby steps.

The hundreds of patients I have worked with who have made the incredible changes in their bodies from dysfunctional— or in some cases almost nonfunctional—to optimal have been the ones who have said: *I am ready. Enough is enough already. I am ready to take that first baby step.*

One popular definition of insanity is doing the same thing over and over, expecting different results. Most of us are guilty of having done this to some extent. If you keep doing the same things, your path will remain the same; your life can't change and your health will remain the same.

The truth is that in order for things to change, *we* need to change; in order for things to happen, *we* need to make them happen. The people who understand this are the ones who are able to move forward and get results.

Choosing to Change

Will H. was a supermarket clerk, a stocker in a large store. He was sixty-four when he came to see me. He had been at one of our dinner seminars and was struck to find out that many of the issues that he had were potentially reversible because he had never thought about it like that. He was obese; he had diabetes with nerve damage to his feet. He had injuries from previous accidents, and he had so much pain in his legs that he was no longer able to walk up and down the aisles of the large store he worked. He was three years away from retirement and at risk of losing his whole retirement package if he couldn't stay at work. His boss was unwilling to give him a less physical job, so he was really stuck.

Will had attended the dinner talk with his brother, who was physically in a similar condition but was retired. His brother chose not to engage in changing his health. Will jumped into his program and was a very good student. Within a few months, he had lost more than thirty-five pounds, and his pain levels went down significantly. Also, his nerve pain began to get better, his energy improved tremendously, and he was able to increase both his stamina and his strength at work.

He graduated the program after six months. I ran into him about twelve months later. He came into our office to tell us that people couldn't believe how active he was and how well he was doing. He was excited to tell us that he was able to do his job with complete ease, and he was enjoying life so much more because of what he was now able to do.

On a sad note he told us that he had just buried his brother three weeks before—his brother, who had chosen not to make any changes in his health, had a severe stroke and Will took care of him until he passed away. He told us that he had so wished that his brother had had the motivation to make the necessary changes in his health, as he might still be alive. Will was grateful that he himself had gotten well enough to be able to give care to his brother in the end when his brother could not take care of himself.

So, he said, "I was working full time and taking care of my brother. And I was able to do it."

WHERE DO YOU SEE YOURSELF IN FIVE YEARS?

Where do you see yourself in the future?

What can you see when you look ahead five years?

When I ask my patients these questions, they have a variety of responses. Some of them see themselves dead in three to five years. Others see themselves as disabled and unable to care for themselves anymore. Some see themselves as being more dependent on others. Others say they see themselves as being more isolated, unable to go out as much, or travel as often, unable to interact with their families and friends as much or do the things they want to do.

Your Future Is Up to You

I invite you to take a moment to sit down, get comfortable, take three nice, slow, deep clearing breaths, close your eyes—if it feels comfortable—and try to visualize how you see yourself in five years with your current trajectory of health. It will only take a few minutes.

Here are some questions to consider:

- Where do you see yourself?
- What are your abilities?
- What kinds of things are you doing?
- Are you working?
- Are you traveling?
- Are you spending time with your family and friends?
- Are you socializing a lot with your friends?
- Are you giving back to your community?
- Where do you see yourself?
- Are you limited by the fact that your body doesn't feel well?
- Are you limited by your foggy brain?
- Are you limited by your fatigue?
- Are you limited by your chronic gut issues?

- Are you limited by your pain?
- If nothing changes, how do you see yourself in three to five years?

Now, let's say you receive the help that you need and make some lifestyle changes that maybe you needed to make. Let's say that it's now three to five years later, and you're right where you want to be. Now think about it. Feel about it.

What do you envision?

Where do you see yourself?

What do you see yourself doing?

What would you do if your body, your mind, your emotions, and your spirit were all working just how you wanted them to be?

What would your life look like?

The Choice Is Yours

You can stay on your current trajectory, or you can join the thousands of people before you who took their lives into their own hands and turned their health around.

Really, for the most part, the choice is yours. Many of the things that are not working in your body can be changed if you make that choice.

Consider what your trajectory looks like.

Where are you heading?

Are you going to keep that trajectory?

If your choice is yes, that choice is to be honored and respected.

But if your choice is to join the thousands of people before you who have decided to start with those baby steps and then maybe take bigger steps and actually see how optimally their bodies can function, given some relatively small changes, wouldn't that be exciting?

You have this choice. It is completely your choice. Nobody can make this choice for you. Nobody can tell you that now is the time or now is not the time. Nobody can decide for you that your better health is worth the investment of your time and commitment and finances. You are the only one who can make this choice. You are in charge.

My Hope for You

I have had the honor of watching thousands of people choose *yes* and embark on the path to change. I have been able to witness the incredible life changes that so many of my patients have made.

On a weekly basis, I get to sit with people who are talking about change they never even thought possible, healing their bodies and their lives.

Now, my hope for you is that you sit with this choice, acknowledge the importance of this choice, and ultimately make the choice to begin—right here, right now—on your journey toward healing. So much is possible. I hope that someday I can celebrate your incredible accomplishments with you.

From Desk Potato to the Camino Trail!

Jane, seventy, came in as a self-described *desk potato*. She was just finishing up a very stressful desk-based career. She described herself as going from desk to couch, exhausted all of the time, fifty pounds overweight, and addicted to carbs. She had never exercised a day in her life. Her brain was completely foggy, and she was concerned about early dementia.

Jane's lab tests revealed high levels of inflammation, pre-diabetes, and elevated cholesterol. After just a few weeks of correcting underlying dysfunctions, addition of missing nutrients, and changes in food choices, Jane's head started to clear. She had more energy and wanted to start moving her body. She started at a gym and found that she loved it so much she started going almost daily. Her brain, energy, and mood began to spiral upward, and her weight started melting off. Six months later, Jane is fifty pounds lighter and training to hike the El Camino trail in Spain in a few months. She is amazed every day at her new abilities and at how young she feels!

Testimonials

I am feeling better than I have in years—sleeping deeply, reducing belly fat and bloating, and my acid reflux has been alleviated! I also have less anxiety and more energy—so many issues I didn't even know I was experiencing until they were gone. Also, when I started the program, I was six weeks away from knee replacement surgery. Four weeks in I was no longer having any knee pain despite working a full day in my garden! My orthopedic surgeon suggested that we don't even need a visit for another year!

~ Linda Marr, 73

The biggest parts of the success of this program is Dr. Laura's passion and interest in every person and her excitement and energy. Joining a group that cares about you and makes you feel at home and you have a lot of support. It's not easy but it's wonderful! It's been a really fun and happy part of my life.

~ Valerie Sauve, 65

Better memory, better eating, better sleep, better . . . well, better everything.

~ Gary Beall, 74, and Sharon D. Smith, 76

Conclusion

I hope that after reading this book, you now see that there is an in-depth, logical, practical, and smart way to look at your body and figure out what is going on.

What is making you feel unwell?

How can you feel better?

Answering these questions is not a matter of magic; it's a matter of smart science, paying attention, and digging deep. There is a logical, practical way to turn a lot of these problems around. My work and the work of hundreds of other doctors around the world have shown us that much of what ails us can be helped. With that said, the change comes only if you are willing to take the steps needed to make it happen.

We have been trained by modern medicine to expect to go to our doctor and get a treatment—usually some kind of pill that takes our problems away. These days are over. The days of the magic pill are over. The magic pills that we get from our doctors may make us feel better temporarily, but most of the time, they are not changing the course of our health issues at all. In the long run, they don't get us to a better place.

You have the ability to turn the trajectory of your health and to give your body what it needs to function optimally. Much of what prematurely kills us or disables us is both preventable and reversible. Turning it around is completely within your control and up to you.

If you do nothing else, I urge you to at least talk to a doctor who specializes in searching for the root causes of your health issues to learn what you can do to turn your health issues around. Many of these doctors, myself included, consider themselves a part of the growing field of what is becoming more commonly referred to as *Functional Medicine,* or root-cause medicine. When you receive help from someone who can assess your state of health and let you know what you can do about it, then you will be empowered to take that first step.

Taking care of yourself is your choice. Most of us, unfortunately, take better care of our cars than we do our bodies. We are each given one body in this life; this physical body is needed to get us through each day and each moment in our lives. If you ignore your body when it is asking for help, eventually it is going to stop allowing you to use it the way you want to. If you pay attention, you can help it get to where you need to go.

It is your choice. You have the power. The knowledge and assistance are out there.

It may be a bit of an investment of time and money, but what is your time and money worth if you don't have a working body to enjoy it?

I hope you make the choice that hundreds of my patients have made: to invest in your own health and get to the bottom of what is making you sick. You can join my patients in seeing what is truly possible for your body and your brain. It is my hope that you find a way to change the trajectory of your health and get the most out of your life.

My team offers an introductory seminar to outline how we can help you. Our expertise is not only in our *root-cause* approach, but also in giving you the support and structure that are critical to making change FOR REAL and FOR GOOD. I encourage you to come to one of my dinner seminars or watching an online webinar and see for yourself what is possible or call my office and speak to one of my team members about what we do.

Explore the options. Help is out there, and you can do it. You have the power to heal much of what ails you. Empower yourself to take action and make it happen. Get your health back.

And what happened to Jeff? Our *root-cause* approach found a combination of gut imbalances, hormone imbalances, inflammation, and nutrient deficiencies. Within a few months, Jeff was completely back on top of his game. His energy and moods were great, his brain was sharp again, and his muscle-to-fat ratios were back to a healthy place. Most importantly, his relationships with his wife and family improved, and he was back to fully enjoying life. He got his MOJO back!

> *What I, as an engineer, like about Rosa Transformational Health is the root cause approach. Going back to what is causing the problem and not just treating with pills.*
>
> ~ Jim Anderson, 83, Engineer

Next Steps

You are invited to learn more about how we can help you turn your health around and achieve your health goals.

Call our Transformation HOTLINE at 541-816-4336 to learn more or to sign up for a FREE Informational Dinner Seminar or Online Webinar.

> *I recently turned 40 and have been overweight for 30 of those years! I have had many years of stress, depression, anxiety, chronic pain, anemia, insulin resistance, weight gain, and a tiredness that bordered on lethargy. I was fed up with how awful I felt! The Rosa program has changed my life in so many ways. I quickly had no pain, lost weight, and reversed my depression. Now my energy is great and my blood work is continually improving! I have tools to reduce my stress. I am finally looking forward to the next 20 years and more!! Thank you, Rosa!!*
> ~ Kari Duran, 40

> *I started the program because my mobility was so limited I was going to apply for a handicap permit. Now I am getting my bicycle tuned up so I can ride with friends. As a bonus, I have lost almost 30 lbs and the weight is still dropping.*
> ~ Laura Hemingway, 61

I feel free as a butterfly is after it's changed from a crawling caterpillar. I was like that crawling caterpillar grounded with many ailments. Rosa wrapped me in their caring, knowledgeable cocoon, and now I am free and healthy. I was obese, my diabetes was out of control causing stage III kidney failure. I had asthma and sinusitis, heart failure, high cholesterol, high blood pressure, had low energy, and felt sick all the time. I was taking 17 prescriptions (with no marked improvement). Dr. Laura and the staff at Rosa offered a caring, knowledgeable plan and listened to me. I am no longer obese, my diabetes is under control, cholesterol and blood pressure are good for my age. Now I only take 4 prescription drugs! I have stamina and energy. Instead of staying in bed all day, I am up working outside non-stop!

~ Herb Ocobock, 77 years old, feel like 66!

About the Author

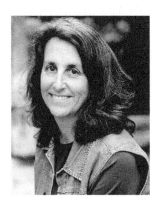

Dr. Laura Robin co-founded Rosa Transformational Health in Medford, Oregon, with Dr. Mona Tara in 2015. Dr. Robin graduated from the Philadelphia College of Osteopathic Medicine in 1988 and completed a residency and Masters in Public Health at the Johns Hopkins Bloomberg School of Public Health in 1993. She completed further training as a Medical Epidemiologist through the U.S. Centers for Disease Control's Epidemic Intelligence Service. She maintains board certification in Family Practice, Public Health and Preventive Medicine, and Integrative Holistic Medicine.

For nine years, Dr. Robin had a private practice in Integrative Medicine in Bend, Oregon. For ten years, she served as the Medical Director of the Student Health and Wellness

Center at Southern Oregon University in Ashland and served as its co-director from 2012–2015. She served on the Jackson County Medical Advisory Board and the Jackson County Public Health Advisory Board. She lives in Ashland, Oregon, with her son, Ari.

Made in the USA
Monee, IL
15 December 2020

53535149R00075